'Inana
HEALING

'Inana
HEALING

Hawaiian Wellness for Life

Leilani Anderson

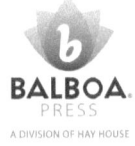

BALBOA
PRESS
A DIVISION OF HAY HOUSE

Inquiries regarding permission for use of the material contained in this book should be addressed to:
'Inana Healing/CareshiftersTM Healthy Aging Institute
P.O. Box 600144
Dallas, Texas 75360
214-755-0213

Balboa Press books may be ordered through booksellers or by contacting:

Balboa Press
A Division of Hay House
1663 Liberty Drive
Bloomington, IN 47403
www.balboapress.com
1-(877) 407-4847

Because of the dynamic nature of the Internet, any web addresses or links contained in this book may have changed since publication and may no longer be valid. The views expressed in this work are solely those of the author and do not necessarily reflect the views of the publisher, and the publisher hereby disclaims any responsibility for them.

The author of this book does not dispense medical advice or prescribe the use of any technique as a form of treatment for physical, emotional, or medical problems without the advice of a physician, either directly or indirectly. The intent of the author is only to offer information of a general nature to help you in your quest for emotional and spiritual well-being. In the event you use any of the information in this book for yourself, which is your constitutional right, the author and the publisher assume no responsibility for your actions.

Any people depicted in stock imagery provided by Thinkstock are models, and such images are being used for illustrative purposes only.
Certain stock imagery © Thinkstock.

ISBN: 978-1-4525-3337-7 (sc)
ISBN: 978-1-4525-3338-4 (e)

Library of Congress Control Number: 2011924252

Printed in the United States of America

Balboa Press rev. date: 4/15/2011

Dedication

After twenty years of study and mentorship
with my kumu- and beloved Tutu, she gave
me her blessing of Aloha as a practitioner
of the Hawaiian Healing Arts.

'Inana Healing is dedicated to her wisdom,
strength, and vision of an evolved society,
brimming with vitality and purpose.

Tutu Violet Ku'ulei Kahale Bourke

1919-2010

Acknowledgements

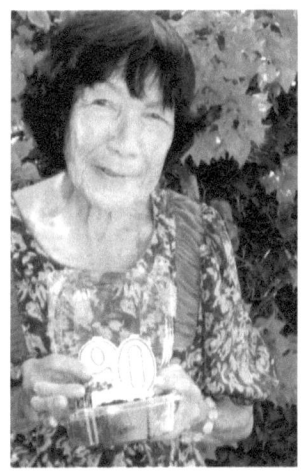

I would like to give thanks and love to my Tutu's children, Marlene Bourke-Faustina, and Patrick Bourke.

Marlene is the grand-daughter of Rose Campbell, Lady-In-Waiting and Royal Court Dancer for the late Hawaiian Monarch, Queen Lydia Lili'uokalani. Marlene has devoted her royal education to the arts, serving as an accomplished performer and master educator in the Hawaiian tradition. A lead soloist with the Royal Hawaiian Band, she was gifted in portraying heartfelt, authentic interpretations of Hawaiian life and culture. Marlene continues to apply the meticulous elements of hula, song, language, and handicrafts into panoramic expression.

Patrick, grandson of Rose Campbell, devoted his royal legacy to Alaka'i, or Leadership, modeling the Hawaiian virtues of respect, honesty, and humility as a Major in the United States Air Force. Patrick has spent his life honoring his culture through daily word and deeds, sharing the spirit of Aloha with family, colleagues, and friends. My father, Patrick, embodies the essence of *Ho'opono Pono Ke Ala*, providing the tone and character of this book.

Mahalo Nui Loa, Marlene and Patrick, for sharing these gifts with my family.

Contents

Summary

I believe that ultimate prosperity lies in the creation and maintenance of owning and earning vibrant, lasting health, and is worth more than any treasure on Earth.

It is my hope that the ancient principles and practical applications researched for this book will encourage you to reflect, transform, and mentor others in the areas of mental, physical, spiritual, and psychic wellness.

May your journey in ultimate prosperity not only become a privilege, but a birthright!

Mahalo Nui Loa,
Leilani

Introduction

In ancient Hawaiian tradition, the creation and maintenance of optimal health demonstrated a divine gift. This gift was led by a healer, or (kahuna), and supported by everyone in the village. Optimal Health connected the village directly to the divine, where blessings were offered, and prosperity was measured. Any illness that existed in the village noted a disconnection with the divine, putting the power of its' people in question. Daily access and use of massage, herbs, and breathwork eliminated toxins, and renewed the body for the activities of the day. The soul was fortified by a group philosophy (Ho'opono Pono Ke Ala), which practiced ultimate love, forgiveness and extreme acceptance of self and others. As a result, stress and its' related effects did not have a compatible language or environment in which to thrive. This philosophy altered each person on a cellular level, giving the individual power to self-correct any disconnection that existed previously. Offerings of prayer to the divine included only the highest artistic expression, requiring intense mental focus and expertise. Chants in dance and song, weaving bark and botanicals for architecture and crafts, and understanding constellation positions in navigation and sport had to be interpreted with accurate detail. This blend of survival through divine art and intellect was honored through the motto "Ho'olu Lahui", or "Allowing Our People To Flourish". This state of peak performance fed individual purpose and infused a stronger current of energy, happiness, and health in the village. Beginning and ending each day in harmony with mind, body, and soul resulted in a daily renewal, allowing one to "come to life".

In today's health industry, illness and disconnection has provided our society and economy with many unintended rewards. Marketing our lack of divinity, our lack of power, and lack of forgiveness in others has created both an economic and psychic boom for pharmaceutical, psychiatric, and pastoral paternalism. Instead of learning how to develop our power center, our personal gifts and blessings of body, mind, and soul are called into question. Any attempt to strike out against the norm can easily be checked by the enemies of the day. Our modern day villagers foster our insecurities with media gossip, reliance on surface learning, and replacement of conversation with technology devices. A lifestyle that simply exists as a means to an end has choked us off from the divine oxygen needed to thrive in a state of optimal health. For those of us that have been fortunate enough to establish healthy eating, exercise, and relaxation patterns in daily life, our "raison d'etre" may still be unexplored and unexpressed. The idea of flourishing in renaissance, in peak, may have been previously considered a separate goal for specialists in performance technology... but for us? If we already have the power to achieve both optimal health and peak performance FOR LIFE, how can we get there?

'Inana Healing™ was written for this type of health seeker. Unlike contemporary health philosophies and systems, you will learn how to create, develop, and showcase inherent strengths and gifts as a conduit toward higher energy levels, and power for life. Understanding the mystical art and intelligence behind ancient Hawaiian principles provides practical and modern applications in daily living.

'Inana Healing - Hawaiian Wellness for Life endorses this practical approach, teaching you how to harness your energy to maximize your strengths in the creation, design, development, and execution of a Progressive Wellness Environment, or (PWE). Your PWE is your unique passport into your power center, your well of prosperity in terms of vital expression. 'Inana includes health rituals in a variety of forms, used to fortify your (PWE). Massage and meditations in the Hawaiian tradition, Sensory Excursions, and Extreme Adventures are fun activities that allow your confidence and courage to shine, putting your (PWE) into action. Finally, 'Inana designed a T3 (Time, Tact, Talent) approach to give weight, value, and sequence to high impact activities, providing you the necessary tools for living in a state of peak, of renaissance. If we are able to use our inner compass to point toward wholeness in mind, body, and spirit, we have already begun a major internal transformation. Experience the benefits of a revolution in self- empowerment, and connecting with others in the pursuit of optimal wellness. May you remain enthusiastic in your successive health journeys!

Chapter One

'Inana Healing: An Ancient Art Meets Modern Demands

My First Health Journey

Journey in Healing, Take 1

I experienced my first lessons in healing upon meeting my Tutu, Violet Anna Ku'ulei Kahale Bourke. As a child, Tutu was self-disciplined, resourceful, and completely focused on survival. Early experiences of sacrifice and self-preservation allowed my Tutu to ration her energies and resources. This gave way to an independent nature, budding creativity, and spirit of adventure.

She embraced the ancient Hawaiian lifestyle in a modern age, teaching me the timeless interconnectedness of nature, community, and divinity in healthy living. A kahuna, or expert, Tutu Violet specialized in various roles that enhanced relationships, honored existing commitments within her community, and nurtured our relationship from the very beginning, creating my first Hawaiian values. For my first twenty summers, my Tutu traveled 5,000 miles between O'ahu and New York to visit me and my family. Each summer was a celebration, enjoying local food and stories of life on the islands. My first important observation of my Tutu was in her ability to experience life with laughter and an upbeat attitude. Despite an occasional misunderstanding between friends or family, my Tutu was filled with a spontaneous laugh, and had a natural propensity for bringing light to unwell places. A state of natural harmony and well-being created a language rich in detail for poignant memories, and a specific reaction to something joyful could be heard deep in her gut (na'ao), a sign that something expressed was authentic, and could resonate with others in a humorous way.

Working and living with such a joyful heart created an abundance of energy, or mana, between us. This relaxed state of happiness, and joy, is known as hau'oli, and served the ancient Hawaiians well as a cooperative, fun, and sharing community. The benefits of hau'oli energy cleansed and purged imbalances and disharmonies within mind and body, increasing our stores of personal mana. Laughter opened up your lungs, stretched your diaphragm, eased chest tension, and blood vessel function, reduced blood pressure and heart rate, and enhanced blood oxygen levels to promote overall circulation. Living daily in such a fertile environment created a close, long-distance relationship that served us with lasting purpose over the years.

The Hawaiian arts of lomilomi, hula, and handiwork were unique to building health with a vision of beauty, and endorsed my second childhood value in being Hawaiian, Nani.

In ancient times each person from kupuna, grandparent, to keiki, child, received lomilomi massage every day to maintain good health. At the end of the day they would gather together to massage each other, and to talk about what had happened that day. Lomilomi was important for the physical relief it brought, and brought families closer together. Healing of the body was done through massage, and Lau'au'lapa'au, the use of medicinal herbs and plants. Healing of the mind was done through a form of meditation, chant, and prayer. During her summer visits with me, Tutu would practice the healing art of lomilomi massage on her muscles to tone and relax her body before sleeping. As a young child, lomilomi served to help me understand my internal system, and replace patterns of vulnerability for patterns of strength.

Perceived nervousness was nurtured with a blanket of calm, and was an early gift of tactile and spiritual beauty.

Hula, a Hawaiian folkdance, and living history of the Hawaiian people, tells their myths and legends, stories and values through songs, chants and music. Hula is accompanied by dance, descriptive hand gestures and rhythmic movement of feet and hips. As a youth, my Tutu was both a modern dancer and an interpreter of hula, definitely one that learned to listen to her body. She knew exactly when she was not in alignment with others, immediately operating on instinct and intuition. Tutu never had a problem dropping an imbalanced relationship, or cutting off an insincere alliance. She believed her truths to be evident- whether that truth was experienced physically, emotionally, mentally, energetically, or spiritually. In later years, Tutu Violet relied more on peace, poetry, and answers through daily rituals of chants, intricate hand movements, and detailed dance steps. She fueled an inner glow that was revered, protected and shared only with a select few. Fortunately for me, I was one of her select students. As a child, I would watch my Tutu transport herself to another dimension through the beauty of hula. Ancient prayers included recognition, praise, cleansing, forgiveness and request, giving tools to explore creativity and self-care. Nani was expressed in hula by gathering and assembling fragrant, colorful flowers to wear as a necklace, or lei. The materials for the lei worn in Tutu's performances were gathered in her garden, after climbing her plumeria tree for fresh petals. Becoming one with an organic environment revives all Hawaiian ancient art, bringing a renewed sense of purpose and vibrancy.

Tutu seemed to relish her annual summer visits in New York as an ambassador of her Hawaiian heritage, and taught me how to embrace my culture through her example. However, I learned how to adopt her third value, ho'ohana,(or creating one's life purpose), during our absences, and developed this idea into adulthood. My Tutu worked and saved for many years, practicing patience, courage, and creativity to transform her ho'ohana, traveling the world, into a reality. Tutu Violet took the time and effort to fortify her adult education by chronicling a life of exploration. I would live vicariously through her in photographs, strolling along the Great Wall of China, marveling at the masterpieces of Europe, Asia, and The Americas. Tutu would visit five of the seven

'Wonders of the World' in her lifetime, expressing a worldview that made sense with her values and priorities. As a result, she continually re-formulated goals and her vision of life as she achieved each step in her ho'ohana.

Remembering my Hawaiian lessons from childhood, it felt natural to blend these values into a western, modern life purpose, my ho'ohana as a young adult. I viewed health as both tactile and spiritual, simple and mysterious. I spent my visits apart from my Tutu practicing lomilomi, endorsing a healthy diet, and creating artwork as a means to express Nani (beauty), and cultivate mana, (energy). I began my college studies in Psychology and career in mental health concurrently, so I would be able to research and reflect the contrasts of theoretical coursework and practical sessions with real people. In the early stages of my career in mental health, I was trained and focused on healing others from a traditional social work model. I leapt to meet the mental, social, medical, and service needs of my clients, developing programs that reflected their past diagnoses and present challenges, furiously combing any and all existing resources to create future opportunities in achieving total wellness.

Time and again, my best-laid plans were put to the test, as multiple clients would fail to show for appointments, or sit passively in silence, until my "plans" for health and wellness were printed up, documented, and placed in their proper charts. I remember sitting through endless team meetings, listening to similar accounts of well intentioned colleagues, supervisors, and administrators recounting poorly executed communication and care plans from their respective caseloads.

I remember thinking if I only tried a little harder, demonstrated the right attitude and altitude of enthusiasm and strength, that my clients would feed off of my ferocious energy, and decide to become well. Although these may have been necessary conditions for initial success, they were not lasting or sufficient conditions for individual empowerment.

Burned out and totally desperate, I sought much-needed advice on the prospects of health and healing from renowned psychiatrists and health professionals in my field. After shedding many tears of frustration and doubt, I was bluntly informed never to desire a more successful health outcome than the person the successful health outcome was intended for! After seeking guidance from the experts, I felt overwhelmed, foolish, and ill-equipped to meet the challenges of my current post.

I tried to overcome my newly battered self-esteem by spending more time with my clients, colleagues and superiors. I dove into every medical journal and text, researching and asking more and more questions about my current state of wellness! Regarding my training, my natural ability, and my future, I questioned my survival in the roles I would be asked to portray in the field of health and healing. Participating in what I perceived to be a broken system, I felt very much like the clients I spent my waking hours trying to serve. My soul dried up, leaving me empty, disenfranchised, and feeling like an utter failure.

At age twenty, and two years of formal service in the mental health field, I left my job and my undergraduate studies for sunny Waikiki, where I would soon find my greatest health treasure.

For the next twenty years, I became a student of both spiritual and practical lessons in healthy living from my Tutu Violet. In Hawaii, kumu literally means "source". Either through lineage, or lifelong tutelage with a master of a certain craft, you are then honored to practice in the kumu tradition. My Great-Grandmother, Rose Campbell, served as a Royal Court Dancer and a Lady-In-Waiting to the late Queen Lili'uokalani during the final years of her reign.

Great Grandmother Rose passed down the Royal Hawaiian Arts of Hula, Song, and Ho'okipa (Regal Hospitality) to her children and grandchildren, preserving a precious piece of this unique time in history.

My Tutu Violet earned a place in my heart as my first kumu. In my childhood, Tutu provided the 'source', or a foundation for positive, productive thought. Her lessons and annual visits kept us connected through life's general highs and lows, keeping depression, anxiety, and other psychic ills at bay. As a loving grandmother, she had a vested interest in making sure all of her grandchildren remained free of the stressful confines of a modern western health model. Tutu designed a blueprint for physical survival organically rooted in her childhood cultural traditions, and developed this blueprint into a personal wellness plan for her family, reflecting the ancient Hawaiian Healing Arts. Tutu's approach to health and healing was simple, but never easy. This discipline consisted of a daily diet of swimming, eating raw foods through subsistence farming/diving, performing music and dance, creating detailed handicrafts, and maintaining a positive outlook on meditation, massage, and movement. My Tutu Violet rounded out my soul as a warrior and analytic teacher of physical fitness and preventive health, fleshing out a prototype akin to most "boot camps" today.

"It is the right behavior,
conducted at the appropriate time,
by the proper people,
presented to the correct recipients,
toward a positive and significant end."

- Hana Kupono

Upon my first 'adult' visit to Hawai'i, I did everything in my power to put on a brave face, and calmly relay to family and friends that I was going to leave my career and college studies in New York to make a life change on the islands. Finding work and a college transfer proved to be a simple and efficient process; confiding in my Tutu about the details of my silent nervous breakdown were not as easy. For the first two weeks of residency, I could not vocalize how I arrived to her in such a fragile mental state. Instead, I would observe my Tutu in repose, a sustaining example of vibrant physical and mental fitness. During those two weeks, she did not ask what she could do to fix what was wrong with me, and went about the business of living her best life. Shortly afterwards,

I observed changes in my breathing, sleeping, and general mental outlook. Anxiety dissolved, and a feeling of centeredness replaced my former state of confusion. In her absence, I began to feel a familiar, silent blessing, proving to me that the values instilled in me as a child would provide the foundation for a transformation, for life.

Kumu Violet- The Transformation Begins

I spent six months in direct communication with my new 'kumu', without mentioning a word about my recent health crisis. Instead, I developed an incredible appreciation for Violet's daily activities in health, her rituals. I found that her health philosophy was truly from the ancients. Hawaiians lived in a communal society where much of the family possessions were owned by the whole community, though an individual's personal possessions were treated with the greatest respect. But few things were individually owned. The land, the sea and the sky were free for everyone. Violet developed a daily regime of fresh air and sun, walking on the hot sand, climbing trees for plumerias in leimaking, swimming and foraging for limu and opihis (seaweed and mollusk), practicing hula, tai chi, and meditation were spent on Queen's Surf Beach in Waikiki. In ancient times there were two heiau (temples) in this area that covered Queen's Surf. One was Kupalaha, located on the shoreline at Queen's Surf Beach and thought to be part of the Papaíenaíena Heiau, where Kamehameha I made the last human sacrifice in Waikiki. The other, Makahuna, near Diamond Head, was dedicated to Kanaloa, the god of the ocean. I truly believed that performing daily rituals on sacrificial ground blessed and fortified Violet, and became her religion, since she saw divinity as an abundant provider of her needs. Once the sun set, Violet meditated, gave pause to the arts and messages of health that she practiced during the day. She operated within her frame of reference to develop her strengths, thrived in the construction of a progressive wellness environment. During my stay in Hawai'i, I learned not only the mystical, aesthetic aspects of health and healing, but absorbed Violet's discrete, pragmatic advice that I would practice for life.

Kumu Violet's Evening Meditations

1. Exercise Regularly: This one may seem obvious but it needs to explained. Regular exercise not only keeps your muscles working but it also releases endorphins into your bloodstream, making you feel good. Regular practice continuously develops the muscle memory that you need for optimal health. Taking small breaks to recuperate through the breath, or 'ha', promotes relaxation is an important part of regular exercise.

2. Eat Raw Foods: If you eat raw foods then your body will function better. Fresh fruit, seaweed, fish, and coconut milk supplies magnesium, amino acids, and live minerals, giving the energy you need to function optimally.

3. Practice of the 'Ha" Deep Breathing: Practicing 'ha' breathing is not only a great way to get relief from stress, but it also supplies oxygen to the blood, bones, and brain. Lung strength helps endurance in all activities, and improves concentration.

4. Do Visualizations: Apply natural settings in meditation to enhance the effectiveness of your visualization, as it takes you to a deeper level of mind. Meditation combined with visualization will improve your concentration and focus as well has improving your flow of daily activities.

5. Stay Positive: Keeping a positive attitude and mind set is essential for peak performance. Keep yourself surrounded by a feeling of Aloha, love, positive people and situations as much as possible.

6. Set Goals: Setting a goal not only focuses the mind, but it also creates a sense of accomplishment once the goal is attained. Setting short-term and long-term goals is the best way to keep yourself motivated.

On the last day of my visit, my kumu settled with me over lunch, positioning questions that would bring me on a lifelong journey to greater heights of health, joy, and purpose:

What do you want to accomplish, and how do you want to get there?

Do you have a plan and system for achieving this process?

How will you use your culture to provide strength in times of need? When will you fight for health? How will you continue to use the gift of health as your power center?

How will you serve others through the gifts of your ancestors? How will you pass on your legacy?

Ultimately, Violet was a person who never lived in the clouds. She understood that I had to learn the basics of health, so I could return to the development of my life's purpose, my ho'ohana. I stayed in Hawai'i for six months, before returning to New York to finish my college studies, and determine the course of my career as a gerontologist and public health advocate.

For the next twenty years, I would remain in close contact with my Tutu, creating an intimate link to her legacy of healing. I truly believe my mental collapse was a blessing, and I was able to honor my ancestors' simple request to listen and absorb life's beauty in a new way. I have taken heed to this request, and have never looked back. We do live in a state of unlimited beauty and power. It is easier take full advantage of this abundant state when one is able to enjoy lasting, optimal health.

I felt extremely fortunate to be the grand-daughter of such a strong and beautiful force of nature. 'Inana Healing was born after Violet's passing, at the sage age of 90, when she found ultimate paradise in peaceful sleep.

Chapter Two

Nourishing a New You

"Nana i ke kumu", advises a famous Hawaiian proverb, "Pay attention to the source."

I had the gift of a loving family member and teacher to show me how to benefit from ancient Hawaiian healing arts and practices, and apply these principles to my health regime. Healing is dependent on the imagination and mindset that release one from the bondage of resentment and judgment. This is the method steeped in traditional Hawaiian Spirituality, and within the ancient teachings identified as Ho'opono Pono Ke Ala – "making right, more right, the path."

Choosing to accept "wellness" at the onset of any health imbalance could generate a subliminal current, suggesting that everyone is making an approximation toward the end goal of wholeness. Ho'opono Pono Ke Ala was a mindset used by health specialists as a precursor to treatment via herbs, massage, prayer, and setting of the bones. This form of ancient healing existed prior to western and missionary influences, and is an unfamiliar practice by most Hawaiians today.

I was fortunate to come from a family that studied and absorbed many practices of Hawaiian culture. In reality, this took some sacrifice on the part of my grandparents, father, aunt, and cousins, especially after the Hawaiian Monarchy was overthrown in 1893. On the islands, assimilation to western lifestyles, annexation, world war, statehood, and technological progress have left the lure of ancient practices to many artists, scholars, and athletes. This focused interest has developed such industries, enriching the lives of many who live in Hawai'i and beyond. What is surprising for many who explore the philosophy of all Hawaiian traditions is the common thread of health as the cornerstone of progress and evolution for its' people.

To ancient Hawaiians, mana (spiritual power) was necessary to be a truly successful practitioner. Hawaiians embrace the family as the basic unit of society and the highest form of human expression, and readily reject the modern ideal of individualism so highly valued in western societies. Hawaiians also hold and use land and water in a collective form rather than a private property form, and to prescribe to the notion and the value that one person should not strive to surpass and therefore outshine all others. By fulfilling their duties to the family and recognizing the accomplishments of others, Hawaiians increase their mana, or spirituality. Education was sacred as knowledge was a way of achieving this power. If a parent sensed a child had a "healing spirit" enabling them to become a doctor, the child would be sent to live and study with a kahuna from as young as five years of age and they would spend upwards of fifteen to twenty years in training. During this time they studied anatomy, learned how to diagnose disease, how to choose the right cures or medicines (particularly the use of medicinal plants), and learned sacred prayers. They also learned how to perform simple surgical procedures, set bones and perform autopsies. Since the Hawaiians viewed the body, mind and spirit as one, Hawaiians believed that the body could not be healed without healing the spirit. Accordingly, they used a combination of psychic, spiritual, and natural treatments to cure illnesses. Kahuna haha diagnosed illnesses by feeling with the fingers. Kahuna hoohanau keiki delivered babies. Kahuna hoohapai keiki induced pregnancy. Kahuna laau lapaau who treated patients with herbs; they were the general practitioners. Kahuna lomilomi who were physical therapists and also skilled in massage. A notable and enduring aspect of Hawaiian Healing in the Ancient tradition is in its' communal focus toward balance and health for everyone. One person that lived out of balance could rest in the knowledge that an entire village was working toward restoration of that balance. That alone provided comfort and accelerated mental powers to self-heal. A more significant and educational facet of the ancients is in its' united front to love the self as a extension of the divine, while remaining humble and helpful to others. This belief eliminated anxiety, depression, confusion, and spite toward self and others. There was a higher sense of respect for cultivating a divine relationship, rather than indulging in power struggles amongst each other. As a result, the concept of "stress" did not have a viable language in which to thrive. Living without such negative influences made it easier for kahuna to diagnose and heal any imbalances within the village.

Healing Rituals

"Understanding exactly how a Hawaiian healer transforms a person would be like asking how you would feel if you were soaked to the bone, shivering, and locked outside your door. You would see yourself outside your home, and let yourself in immediately with a change of clothes, straight from the dryer. You would light a fire, gather blankets, and prepare a hot cup of tea. You would prepare to stay up all night listening, encouraging, and excavating the years of cold, wet, and heavy emotions, replacing them with laughter, light, and soft eyes. By sunrise, you are refreshed, full, and ready to journey into the beyond."

-Quote, K.A.

Healing treatments were used amongst the Hawaiians to initiate and continue a divine relationship with nature. Similar to a physician visit, the kahuna, or specialist of the village would diagnose illness and imbalance in a 'patient' through breath, palpation, observation, and massage. A Kahuna haha was a specialist who diagnosed illnesses by feeling with the fingers. Kahuna lomilomi who were physical therapists and also skilled in massage. Infants, children, adults, and elders all experienced a primary benefit from this relationship, in the form of touch. Sensing immediate comfort upon a kahuna's initial touch often accelerated the restoration process immediately. Contrast your initial feeling upon visiting any western primary physician! The pule, or blessing from the divine would be in the skilled hands of the village's kahunas, who specialized in the prevention and restoration of mana- of energetically based health. Healing and restoration of mana not only helped the person receiving a lomilomi treatment, but positively affected those involved with that person. In ancient tradition, practicing compassion, providing blessings, and supporting one another elevated the consciousness of the entire community.

Today, lomilomi massage and related treatments are internationally recognized in spas, resorts, and healing centers in an effort to revive the ancient philosophy of our kahunas.

Receiving a modern lomilomi treatment is a unique way to fortify and fine tune your goals and objectives, as you transform your intentions into a systematic, integrated health model. Eliminating mental, physical, and spiritual toxins through breath work, or (Ha), clears the body of congestion and increases oxygen to the organs. Healing from the inside is administered through the art of the blessing, or pule. A pule may be done silently, or through chant while the external body is treated. The skin is brushed and purified with salt, botanicals, and oils in preparation for the massage, as muscle and tissues are kneaded to increase circulation and range of motion to the external body.

A final pule is given as a lasting transmission of love, forgiveness, and expectation for unity between the internal and external realms. This provides a springboard for growth, and an increased awareness of the path you are on, in terms of sustaining optimal health.

Living in peace, treating health as one's ultimate currency has given me pause many a time when applying my Hawaiian Health values to modern day living. I have found this to be a personal struggle without fortifying the power of the mind, "Ho'oulu Lahui".

Chapter 3

Adopting Your Role- "Hou'olu Lahui"

Archaeological evidence indicates the Hawaiian islands were well populated by A.D. 500, but the first settlers may have arrived several centuries earlier. Wood, stone, bone, fibers and feathers were the artisans' primary materials. The early Western explorers found the Hawaiian artistic traditions closely linked to the ancient religion of Hawaii. Dance, music and arts celebrated the elements, gods and human abilities. Congress defines "Native Hawaiian" as "any individual who is a descendant of the aboriginal people who, prior to 1778, occupied and exercised sovereignty in the area that now constitutes the State of Hawaii." (U.S. Public Law 103-150) Today the maka'ainana, the artisans, carry forth the creative legacy of their ancestors who traveled far across the seas from legendary Havaiki, islands not anchored in any ocean-the home of all knowledge. Ancient Hawaiian values faded over time, with each successive reign. Kapu, or forbidden practices were, in part, established to protect sovereign power. International influences from foreign explorers created a significant cultural disintegration within villages, creating psychic chaos and despair - for the first time in Hawaiian history.

King David Kalakaua (1874–1891) was a visionary on many fronts, namely because he sought to revive Ancient Hawaiian Arts and Philosophies not only for his people, but for those around to world to marvel and reconnect within this unique culture. King David coined the phrase, "Ho'oulu Lahui", or to "Let The People Flourish".

Many years ago, Ritual and prayer surrounded all aspects of Hawaiian training and practice, from the musical arts of hula and song, to the visual stunning pieces displayed for practical use in the musical arts: feather and leimaking, intricate shell and kapa (bark) used for clothing, mats, and adornment. Athletics were also honored and deeply revered in the art of woodcarving. Canoe building from Royal Koa was not only used for sport, but for advanced navigational journeys. Claiming one's divinity through architecture, sport, music, or craft created a haven for those that thrived in the role of a self-healing, divinely connected Emotional Maturity ~ becoming the process of each one that takes on becoming awake in this life. Using this revival as a springboard for evolving through re- creation of Ancient Hawaiian Arts and Culture allowed successive generations to discover and adopt the role of a person in renaissance. This gave tremendous strength, power, and meaning to those affected by previous upheaval and chaos.

Unprecedented international exposure created a legacy for the revival of Hawaiian traditional arts and culture during the reign of King David Kalakaua. He stressed the importance of rediscovering one's heart within the more analytical and competitive mindset of modern day.

Adopting the role of a divine, joyful, intelligent, and expressive person requires some concentration and inner compassion, especially if you are attempting to thrive amongst negative, life-dulling influences. So far, you have learned some basic techniques in self-healing, and how to cultivate your inner resources in nourishing a new, Hawaiian-inspired seeker of joy and vitality. You may have already guessed that necessary and sufficient conditions for health must exist before taking yourself on the more intimate journey of one who exists solely in renaissance, in peak. As you become more successful, there are more pressures and more distractions pulling at you. Harnessing your mana helps you address these distractions, stay focused, and help you continue to sustain your best performances.

In the next chapters, you will find practical tools to harness your mana, using your divine energy to design and implement your Progressive Wellness Environment, or (PWE). This personalized plan will become your coat of arms in attaining a life in the peak state.

Chapter Four

New Energy, New Environment

For our ancestors and modern day health seekers, the Ancient Hawaiian Healing Arts are timeless. Designed to provide you with the divine right to enjoy optimal health, this gift is the highest expression of love and power from the Universe. Your job is to understand how to harness and cultivate your mana, or divine energy, through a study of both internal and external health influences.

The internal discipline required to achieve and maintain a state of lifelong health requires daily practice of Ho' Oponopono Ke Ala. This practice is characterized by one's ability to achieve and maintain a state of extreme love, acceptance, and forgiveness of past transgressions- for self, for others.

This practice showcases both the mystic and analytical elements present in the Hawaiian Healing Arts.

Ho'Oponopono Ke Ala, the primary tenet of Hawaiian Healing, is sometimes perceived as a mystical ability. In ancient Hawaiian culture, placing one's trust in the divine to restore a health balance assumes an acceptance of a structure, a design that is supported by both island life (land, water, flora/fauna) and inhabitants of the island (radical belief and acceptance of healing). An aggressive campaign to restore the individual is a primary goal of the group, understanding that communal health and vitality is the currency and power center for progress of its' inhabitants. The concept of practicing radical self-acceptance, love, objectivity, and stillness in the midst of a health disconnect seems counterintuitive to western health philosophies and practices.

Consider the everyday example of a person who has experienced extreme anxiety over a prolonged period, and who seeks relief from this agitated state. The person sees a physician, describes one's symptoms, and is given a prescription to alleviate those symptoms. Taking a prescription to alter brain chemistry toward a reduced anxiety state takes care of the necessary conditions in promoting mental health. However, one's feelings surrounding the diagnosis, the potential side effects of the prescription, and the afterlife of the treatment fail to supply the sufficient conditions for a restoration, a health balance for the person experiencing the anxious state. As a result, this person runs the risk of duplicating or creating more intense states of anxiety, creating a further disconnect and link to healing power.

Converting health and wellness toward a human ecology model takes "going green" to a whole new level!

Understanding the ancient belief systems of Hawaiian Healing is primarily the ease in which one can adopt a restorative mindset in today's world. Practicing a daily ten minute journey can start the process of living in peace, enjoying Ho' Oponopono Ke Ala.

Meditation Journey for Ho' Oponopono Ke Ala

Guided imagery has been used for centuries to initiate deep breathing, relaxation, and preparation for the mind to manage stressful situations. Your journeys will be based on actual and/or created experiences and observations of Hawaiian landmarks and images to take you away from your everyday irritants, or chronic stressors. If you have never visited the Hawaiian islands, take some time to visit your local bookstore or computer search engine to give your imagination a boost. First, the breath, or Ha, will provide oxygen to the body. Breathe in for seven counts. Hold the breath for twenty-eight counts. Exhale for fourteen counts. Continue this cycle for five minutes a day, and graduate to two sessions, ten minutes a day. Remember your multiples of Seven: 7-28-14. A significant benefit of deep Ha is an increased memory retention, a quick burst of energy to the organs, and an easy way to keep extra pounds off the body. For detoxification purposes, daily Ha breathing exhales negative thoughts, anxiety, and other destabilizing emotions, creating an environment where this destabilization fails to gather strength, power, or meaning. Therefore, stress is not an enemy, because the concept is routinely rejected in favor of the stabilized, harmonious state of health. You are creating a personal and collective environment where stress is unable to find a happy home. So far, you have already discovered how Ancient Hawaiians have specialized in the prevention of disease, and restoration of one's natural balance. You have also learned how to take on the role of a self-healer, flourishing in the powers of mental discipline and increased creativity. "Hou'olu Lahui", the idea that you were destined to express yourself in an ongoing state of peak performance accepts this evolved mind through preparation, energy work, honed strengths, and proper execution of your Progressive Wellness Environment (PWE).

Understanding your 'readiness' before such a transformation takes place is a mysterious concept for even the most confident health seeker. Asking yourself to dissolve ties to people, events, and ideas that do not complement your new Progressive

Wellness Environment (PWE) will be an adjustment for many, especially if such ties served you well in some aspects. For the ancients, a transitional stage from intention to action was often solidified in the space of a lomilomi treatment. Through the kahuna lomi, fingers would "speak to the tissue", providing light to congested areas through varied tones and timbres. Musings, suggestions, and frank admissions to an existing health hunch may appear in a whisper, or expose itself in a loud roar! Either way your body will force you to listen on a deeper level, for you have unique toxins that reside in what may have been a very convenient environment over the years. Take time to have these "final conversations" with your congested places, before stepping out into a new existence of illumination and vibrant thought. Enjoy the panoramic scope of your new life, while healing in the ancient lomi tradition. Take advantage of the simpler methods to healing, and let a treatment wash over you, as you prepare to create your Progressive Wellness Environment!

'Inana Healing Pakolea Lomi- Massage Therapy Treatments

Noho ali'i Massage

This massage pays proper respect to our core posture and back strength. The convenience of an upright position helps target specific muscle groups. A moist heat pack is added to the lower back to aid in your flexibility and strengthening.

'Aki Aloha

This massage treatment assists in relieving chronic headaches, sinus congestion, and neck tension while you enjoy a targeted treatment from the pressures of daily commutes, environmental fluctuations, and general stressors from the outside world.

Lomi Lomi Restorative Exfoliant and Massage

This ancient Hawaiian art form will allow you to enjoy from the inside out. Fresh banana leaves and sea salt are applied to the body, revealing a new glow to the skin. Coconut oil is then applied during this invigorating massage, nourishing the new you. Soothing Polynesian sounds will guide you to relaxation as a pule, or blessing is released to restore the body toward its' optimal state- peace and health.

Loku'u Massage

Loku'u 'Anapu'u, also known as lymphatic drainage, is a gentle, yet effective form of massage that stimulates the lymphatic system to improve metabolism, promote the removal of bodily toxins and waste, and encourages a healthy immune system.

Lani Kua

This massage treatment honors our most precious tools for mobility and balance- our hands and feet. Heated sand and stones immerse both hands and feet, and initiates a series of acupressure, reflexology, and stretching techniques to your muscles, joints, and arches. Ideal for increasing circulation to the body, and relieving stress to overworked extremities.

Pumehana Pule

This unique massage treatment is designed to bring Ho'opono Pono Ke Ala, or balance to the body, mind, and spirit. Using heated lava stones and warmed macadamia oil, long, soothing strokes are applied to the muscles- designed to renew body and soul.

'Ana'Anai Body and Scalp Duet

This delicious signature treatment uses pure macadamia nut oil, raw cane sugar, and guava fruit to exfoliate and polish the body. While the 'anai nourishes the skin, a plumeria and jasmine infused scalp massage will leave you in a state of pure paradise.

Variations of lomi treatments were passed down from my family, generation to generation. The lomi treatments in this book were designed by yours truly, and may not be found in most commercial spas and resorts presently. Not all treatments share identical technical elements, but rather embrace universal intentions for health. Disconnection of mana, or divine energy, is the universal diagnosis. Harmony with the divine, and restoration of mana is the universal cure. Styles and sequence are sometimes dictated by the needs of the recipient, whether you are an athlete, or visiting a state of rehabilitation.

Self healing in the lomilomi tradition is truly attainable, with a bit of imagination and color. If you are already a fan of the Hawaiian aesthetic, you may enjoy a shopping trip to your local health food store to purchase most of your basic lomilomi supplies. Coconut oil, salt, banana leaves, and essential oil creates a basic scrub to use on the body. I began performing lomilomi on myself as a toddler, and continued practicing on my mother as a youth. The experience was a great deal of fun, and kept me useful in my household.

If you are a parent of a young child (under 100 lbs.), ask your son or daughter to walk on your back, or hamstrings, easing tension and creating a fun environment for your keiki. Using the hands to perform a "chop" to your calves and feet awakens the muscles, and forges a connection between all family members.

I am sure if you have been practicing Ho'oponopono Ke Ala for any length of time, you have already recognized the character of its' energy, and its' impact on daily activities. Belief in healing, and the accompanying breath work to sustain this belief can initially seem like an isolating experience for many. In our modern world, the idea of "energy" is marketed and expressed as a burst of adrenaline, inviting one to get excited, pumped, and turbocharged for action. This method is successful for isolated activities of peak performance, such as winning a championship, composing a speech, or performing a concert for a large crowd.

For the purposes of daily living, the perpetual rhythm of existing from dead stop, to sprint, to dead stop can be exhausting and terrifying for all parties involved. The mana, that will assist you in the development of your (PWE) should feel more like a gradual unfolding, a circle of recyclable energy. This energy will enter the cells, rather than swim around in the atmosphere. This mana will be yours to keep. Remember that your mana, your divine energy, never runs out of steam. Instead, imagine an eternal flame- brighter in some moments, and dimmer in other instances. The wind of external environment may alter the strength of the flame, but trust that it will never extinguish. Managing your external environment can assist you in keeping an even and bright-burning flame. Once you have created your foundation for cultivating and storing mana, take this divine energy to fuse your internal influences with your external environment, and learn how to master the enduring state of panoramic health.

External Environment: Guarding The Flame

Facets of a neutral external environment range from the intimate, (sharing a life with the demands of friends family and loved ones), to the necessary, (career expectations and demands) to the mundane (daily chores, sitting in traffic, paying bills). Other facets of a toxic external environment may comprise of the same factors, but with those factors impinging on your vision of living in Ho' Oponopono Ke Ala and Ho' Oulu Lahui.

A quick way to harness your mana, asking for strength is to consult your Heiau, or your 'Sacred Temple' for guidance. This method is similar to meeting with a 'Board of Directors', a group of trusted imaginary advisors who solely work on your behalf. You can begin your day with a meditation to invoke Ho'Oulu Lahui with an engaged mind, holding a spear outside your sacred temple, prepared for potential thieves that seek to steal your strength. Close your eyes, listen, and feel the vibration in the air as you remain a laser focus on the people, places, and things that seek to steal your mana for their benefit. Limit or eliminate direct contact with these influences until you have a specific plan to reengage and manage acceptable contact with such influences. Imagine your personal kahunas, assisting you in this process with a soft voice, a warm hand on your shoulder, and a courageous push outside of your Heiau to accomplish your goal. Continue your meditation to inhale Ho'Oponopono Ke Ala, forgiving all persons and incidental obstacles to your healing path, and exhale the daily toxins that compromised your ideal health state. Finally, complete your meditation by re-entering your Heiau, your sacred temple, and filling this space with color, light, and sounds that promote peace and relaxation. Begin and end your day with this meditation, and notice how former irritants and potential enemies keep away from your rich and powerful path to health.

Chapter Five

Analysis of Strengths

<u>Designing and Implementation of Your PWE</u>

<u>'Inana Healing</u> has provided you with basic tools, showing you how to harness your energy to maximize your strengths in the creation, design, development, and execution of a Progressive Wellness Environment, or (PWE).

Combining the qualities of a loving, peaceful mind that endorses the belief in healing with the engaged, renaissance mind enriches the state of optimal health, keeping you vigilant - as you develop a structure in your quest for peak performance.

In Ancient Hawaiian Tradition, kahunas possessed specialties of strength to promote community strengths. Descendants of this community would, in turn, develop those strengths, and pass along unique gifts of talent to future generations to complement the ideas and technology of the day.

Your Progressive Wellness Environment will become your document to defend, amend, and evolve as you reinforce ideals held in the Hawaiian Healing Arts, living in harmony with optimal health as your power center, and state of ultimate currency.

Ingredients of a PWE

Analyzing one's strengths in the Ancient Hawaiian tradition was a primary language for individual and group communication, since competitive influences toward one another were discouraged, and courage was exemplified in one's character. *Huikala* captured the essence of a person's ability to express the divine self in the material world, and brought blessings of health and prosperity for all. The purpose of creating and using a Progressive Wellness Environment is to give yourself and others the gift of Huikala, the opportunity to showcase your divine talents in everyday life.

A Progressive Wellness Environment is intended to bring every aspect of health and wellness into a portfolio for preventive care and expedient healing. Your PWE should make you the sole subject of your intentions for strength in mind, body, and spirit.

In the Ancient Hawaiian Tradition, four healing prototypes of strength and power brought a village together as a cohesive unit.

Kahunas in every village subscribed to a specific prototype in the world of health and healing. The purpose of adopting a strong role was two-fold. One benefit to defining one's role was in promoting a kahuna's access to others in the village. Maintaining rapport, verbally or non-verbally, unified the individual to the group. If one person was out of balance, the group could intuitively search for a kahuna that would communicate healing and restoration with leadership, kindness, and efficiency.

The Four Healing Prototypes

Nurturer (Ho'ohanai): This type of healer was responsible for maintaining peaceful relations, particularly in the areas of childbirth, grave illness, and death. Areas of expertise included midwifery, chant, and keeping company with individuals that needed encouragement and support. Keeping a peaceful, objective countenance brought strength to the group.

Innovator ('Ike Loa): This healer had a primary stake in thinking "outside of the box", particularly in developing solutions to difficult health procedures, or finding expedient methods of collecting data for an individual's health history, and prognosis for continued healing. Keeping and enthusiastic, positive tone inspired individuals and group consciousness.

Messenger (Ho'omau): This healer was responsible for the delivery of recently discovered methods of progress, and unifying the group's philosophy regarding vibrant health and restoration. Keeping the intentions of higher mind, body, and spirit as a primary theme were paramount. Remaining a spokesperson for successive generations maintained a sense of optimism and consistency.

Executor (Ulu Pono): This healer was in charge of adopting the aspects of a nurturer, innovator, and messenger, with the primary responsibility of curing without relapse, of restoring harmony and imbalance.

The executor was either chosen at a young age for demonstrating an inordinate amount of mana, of natural divine power, or chosen after a lengthy apprenticeship with and elder kahuna.

Honing one's healing skill was a constant pursuit in maintaining the highest standards. Challenging existing health practices for advancements in optimal healing were immediately researched, evaluated and supported to further areas of unexplored interest and study.

Using Your PWE for Peak Performance

In designing your PWE, embody each of the roles of the four kahuna prototypes. Nurturing, innovating, publicizing, and executing your desires for growth keeps your vitality at the helm of any potential obstacle. In the course of my studies in Hawaiian Healing, I have been comforted by the wealth of data that supports the powers of peace, love, forgiveness, and detoxification to expedite and maintain a healthy balance in everyday life.

That being said, there are rare instances when one must go to war to fight for one's health. Designing and implementing a battle plan to fortress against the torrents of negative personalities, disappointments in career, or overwhelming burdens in daily life can be enhanced by using elements of Time, Tact, and Talent in daily acts, words, and deeds.

'Inana Healing teaches you to develop a T3 (Time, Tact, Talent) approach to daily activities. This approach gives weight, value, and sequence to high impact activities, providing you the necessary tools for living in a state of peak, of renaissance. A T3 strategy is structured to give your PWE maximum effectiveness, giving a command to the health seeker to properly organize and manage these three resources. Examine the implications of Time, Tact, and Talent mismanagement in everyday life choices. Time can easily waste the development of a talent, and talent can be easily discarded if one fails to employ tact in crucial situations. When designing your PWE, use the strictures of time, the gift of tact, and the divinity of your talents to work to your advantage.

"Where Did The Time Go?"

Time is the great equalizer for all of us, because we are all given 24 hours in every day to accomplish the tasks that lead to goals, that lead to dreams, that lead to legacy. We have little control over our time spent on this Earth, so respecting time in the daily, 24 hour sense becomes a type of currency you can spend wisely, or throw away on toxic people, lost causes, or inanimate objects.

"Wow, Look at the Time!"

Health and Time are close companions, for both carry potential and kinetic energy for all to use properly- or discard without a moment's notice.

We live in a world constantly inundated with countless distractions and temptations, vying to keep our focus on anything but our chosen tasks, goals, dreams, and legacies. Honing our time effectiveness skills with laser precision takes some self-discipline at first, but take heart! Anyone is capable of using Time as an ally instead of an enemy.

Internal and External threats are often left unnoticed, but are indeed responsible for hijacking one's ability to use our 24 hours in day to maximum benefit.

Understanding Your Internal and External Threats to Managing Your Time

In today's modern society, many of us are programmed to coast, to exist on a low-impact trajectory. Living the path of least resistance in the areas of work, recreation, personal relationships, or individual interest has become the norm for several generations of men and women. Internal threats to time management creep in when one is out of touch with the dynamic relationship between mind, body, and soul. Alyxthymia, the state of being that acts as a precursor to illness and imbalance, can gather strength very easily in a low-impact environment. Ennui, apathy, and feelings of depression/anxiety are prone to take root, dictating the bulk of many schedules.

Habitual engagement in low-impact activities also poses the most dangerous internal threat to one's purposeful existence- assigning one to the role of a perpetual spectator. Maintaining inertia in a low-impact lifestyle only rewards a society that undervalues high individual expectations in daily life.

External Threats To Effective Time Management

Undetected internal threats pave the way for the overwhelming flood of external threats that can creep into daily life. Using your time to inhabit the internal role of a spectator can leave you exposed to a new language of persuasive, external threats to keep you in a low-grade existence. The notion of living in the context of peace, joy, vibrant health, evolved thought, and executed deed are often ridiculed by power brokers in the media and those celebrated in popular culture. A substantive diet of television, internet, and other hand-held devices leaves you at high risk for passive leaks into your power center. Remaining a spectator can become addictive, for you are no longer interested in searching for meaning in independent thought or creative expression. The rituals of self-discipline fall away to convenient avenues for more generic and neutered forms of self-expression. Even family and loved ones fall susceptible to this spectator role. If you are ever in doubt, ask a friend, "What's New?". If the familiar reply is a resounding, "Oh, well, you know. Same old, same old!" then it is high time to begin fighting for health in mind, body, and spirit. Becoming a live participant starts to look very real for the seeker of truth and wisdom in peak performance.

The good news for anyone who has been caught exposed to external threats in wasting time, is in the immediate conversion to living your life as a participant in vibrant health. Engaging in high-impact activities is a practice anyone can develop, at any age and stage of life. A person who exercises control over the daily choices in life makes the most significant impact in the enjoyment and preservation of radiant health.

For instance, if you know that you must exercise five out of seven days out of the week to maintain proper weight, strength, and aerobic capacity, you MUST find a consistent time to exercise, and find a tactful way to express this priority to your inner circle. Developing an order to your day extends to the task of food preparation, and finding a consistent time when you are able to gather a fresh menu of fruits and vegetables. Preparing these foods to nourish your body, and enjoying activities that express your strength are related goals that can be monitored in the T3 design. Showcasing your talent, a fit and fortified body, would be executed in the consistent practice of this particular health strategy.

On a more sophisticated level, achieving Ho'oulu Lahui, or an enlightened mind, becomes even more crucial to achieving an existence in the flow, in creative peak.

The power of an evolved mind is unlimited in scope for both the individual health seeker, and the group of participants actively seeking a restoration, a balance in healing.

After developing a mastery of Time management, The second tier of your T3 strategy, Tact, will be the secret weapon you will develop as a health warrior.

Many view tact as an unnecessary "extra" to everyday communication, saving the skill for special occasions in business and personal life. Tact has become so devalued in today's society, that communication between seemingly intelligent people remains littered with frequent interruptions, provoked conflict, and projections of catastrophe. "Brutal Honesty" and "Telling it Like it Is" have become common phrases in today's world, jeopardizing the quality and the magic of non-verbal communication (touch, listening, music, dance) as well as civil, and thoughtful verbal exchanges.

Employing tact in a timely fashion will become your key to negotiating your intentions in fruitful environments, giving you the multiplying effects of self-actualization. Knowing the proper location, time, preparation, and placement of tact creates a higher vibration of energy, of mana between you and your inner circle, giving you the unique opportunity to teach this strategy to others in need.

The third tier of your T3 strategy, Talent, is the culmination of the proficient use of Time and Tact. Divine talents are part of our cells, our personalities, and our souls. Manifesting our divine talent and capitalizing on our gifts, however, takes years of patience, observation, and study.

Understanding the rigor of self- discipline, practicing the rituals of abundant gratitude and humility, devoting apprenticeship to hone skills, and taking responsibility in the transformation from mastered skill to influential gift is a savored journey for those who have treaded the path toward cultivated talent.

Alaka'i, the practice of Leadership, is an Ancient Hawaiian Value that is earned and developed as a result of divine mana exchanged between the prepared leader and the Universe. Talents realized are precious opportunities for growth for individuals and communities alike, as it brings light to dark places at every opportunity. If we can make a collective effort to live in this light, we will be able to gather the courage, the *Koa* required to teach others to lead in wellness and ultimate prosperity.

Working with Exceptional Populations

Sensory Excursions incorporate the skills of meditation, personalized coaching, and Hawaiian Healing Treatments- In the creation and design of your progressive wellness environment. Theory and Practice are emphasized, and 'Inana Healing approaches the design of your Progressive Wellness Plan in context.

Using gradients of sound, intuition, light and tactile enhancements, you will learn how to to increase endurance, master existing skill sets, and improve responses to stress triggers.

Our esteemed groups include:

Indigenous Healers

Indigo Children and Adults

Professional Athletes, Musicians and Performers

Adults and Children with ADD/ADHD, and

Those Living Within the Spectrum

Integrate gifts to achieve peak performance.

'Inana Healing Serves The Healthy Aging Market

Individuals and Companies Team
With A Healthy Aging Specialist.

Used for public speaking engagements and personal high- power meetings, you can create a winning edge in business. Our Specialist will diagnose specific needs in the area of preventive health, training staff and clientele to design and implement the best health practices for your company.

Providing Environmental Enhancements To Work/ Home

Used for a variety of creative and industrial needs, you can fortify mind, body and soul with optimal placement of sound, light, and empowering elements within your sacred space.

Wellness Courses

Used to engage individuals and groups with the benefits of living passionately, and purposefully. Consultation between Coach and Client create an exciting mix... as you design your Powerful Profile, we will help you get there, and stay there.

We promote your Profile through a system of rehearsal, reinforcement, and celebration in real-life scenarios...transforming you to a state of health and renewal.

Extreme Adventures

Used for the rebel, the renegade, the ultimate pioneer... Our Extreme Adventures stimulate intellectual and physical juices, as you create and display your progressive wellness environment in bold relief!

Summary: 'Inana Healing for the Future

I find it ironic that my beloved Tutu has asked me to share the intentions and traditions of my ancestors in the Hawaiian Healing Arts during a time of unprecedented psychic disconnect.

Relying on the lost art of vibrational healing through observation, employed silence, and laying of hands for primary communication, the use of technological supports "for emergencies only" has caused frustration and some bitterness from my emerging social network of peers, colleagues, and younger family members.

Attempting to carry out a holistic health tradition that spans thousands of years is one type of challenge; creating a new vision for peak performance is yet another. It brings me immense joy to see the majority of my work accepted in practice and lifestyle for several niche markets.

International Spas and Resorts have needed to remain competitive with the luxury market in creating an authentic, culturally sensitive spa experience, while remaining cost-effective and results-oriented. Contracting with a Hawaiian Healing Arts Specialist has given this industry a fresh option, while emerging as a pioneer in peak performance milieu.

Children with psychic gifts and learning exceptionalities have taken the initiative in the design and construction of their Sensory Excursions, providing a greater locus of control as emerging members of a new age.

Finally, our current Baby Boom has created ever-increasing numbers of healthy aging collectives, opening the doors to market innovative solutions in optimal health for industry professionals. 'Inana Healing has introduced Careshifters TM Healthy Institute to mobilize our future sages in achieving personal peak performance. It is my hope that you will accept the challenge of deep healing as an individual, and bring that evolved individual out into the world, showcasing your divinity. Restoration of body, mind, and soul allows all of us to practice the divine in the simplest of joys. Taking comfort in the words of the Ancients,

"He puko'a kani 'aina".

(Translation: A coral reef
(hardens/strengthens/transforms into land.)

In their travels around the Pacific, the Hawaiians would pass by many coral heads, which navigators would mark in their memories and pass on to their apprentices. Eventually, they would notice that these small coral heads would grow into a full islands. Recognizing that we would like to be full-blown successes right away, often we must start our journeys with presence and humility- and over time, like a coral head, we will mature and emerge victorious in our individual and collective health pursuits.

Bibliography

Bailey, Simon T. Release Your Brilliance. New York: HarperCollins, 2008.

Bergson, A. , Tuchak, V. Shiatsu- Japanese Pressure Point Massage. Los Angeles: Pinnacle Books, 1976.

Buber, Martin. I and Thou. New York: Simon & Schuster, 1923.

Burton, Humphrey. Leonard Bernstein. New York: Anchor Books, 1995.

Carlson, Richard. Don't Sweat the Small Stuff... and It's All Small Stuff. New York: Hyperion, 1997.

Csikszentmihalyi Mihaly. Flow. New York: Nightingale-Conant, July 2002.

Curtis, Caroline. Stories of Life in Old Hawaii. Honolulu: Kamehameha Schools Press.1998.

Curtis, Caroline. Tales of the Menehune. Honolulu: Kamehameha Schools Press. 1990.

Evans, William, and Rosenberg, Irwin. Biomarkers-The Keys to Prolonging Vitality. New York: Simon & Schuster, 1991.

Fay, Allen, M.D. PQR: Prescription for a Quality Relationship. New York: Simon & Schuster Inc., 1990.

Friedman, Thomas L. The World Is Flat- A Brief History of the Twenty-first Century. New York: Farrar, Straus, and Giroux, 2005.

Henig, Robin. How A Woman Ages-Growing Older: What to Expect and What You Can Do About It. New York: Ballantine Books, 1985.

Huffington, Arianna. On Becoming Fearless. New York: Little, Brown and Company, 2007.

Kitt, Eartha. Rejuvenate!. New York: Scribner Publishing, 2001.

Kouzes, James, and Posner, Barry. The Leadership Challenge. San Francisco: Jossey-Bass Publishers, 1995.

Lee, Ilichi. Brain Wave Vibration. New York: BEST Life Media, 2009

Levey, Joel and Michelle. Living in Balance. New York: MJF Books, 1998.

McGee-Cooper, Ann. You Don't Have to Go Home From Work Exhausted! A Program to Bring Joy, Energy and Balance to Your Life. New York: Bantam Books, 1992.

Murphy, James D. Flawless Execution. New York: HarperCollins Publishers Inc., 2005.

Pachter, Barbara. The Power of Positive Confrontation-The Skills You Need to Know to Handle Conflicts at Work, at Home, and in Life. New York: MJF Books, 2000.

Ramsey, Valerie. Gracefully. New York: McGraw Hill Companies, 2008.

Ray James Arthur, Sivertsen, Linda. Harmonic Wealth: The Secret of Attracting the Life You Want. Carlsbad: Hyperion Books, 2008.

Robbins, Anthony. Awaken The Giant Within. New York: Simon & Schuster, 1992.

Shaw, Robert. Hawaiian Quilt Masterpieces. New York: Hugh Lauter Levin Associates, Inc. 1996.

Sylver, Marshall. Passion, Profit, & Power: Reprogram Your Subconscious Mind to Create the Relationships, Wealth, and Well-Being That You Deserve. New York: Simon & Schuster Inc., 1995.

Tracy, Brian. Thinking Big. New York: Nightingale-Conant, May 2007.

Vithaldas, Y. The Yoga System of Health and Relief From Tension. New York: Bell Publishing Co., 1952.

Warvin, Bill. The Rancho La Puerta Cookbook. New York: Broadway Press, 1998.

Wattles D. Wallace. The Science of Getting Rich. Elizabeth Towne Company, 1910.

Weil, Andrew Dr. Increase Vitality. Boulder, CO: Sounds True/Body & Soul Omnimedia, 2006.

Whiteley, Sharon, Duckworth, Connie, Elliott , Kathy. The Old Girls Network. : Insider Advice for Women Building Businesses in a Man's World. MA: ThirdAge Inc., , 2005.

About the Author

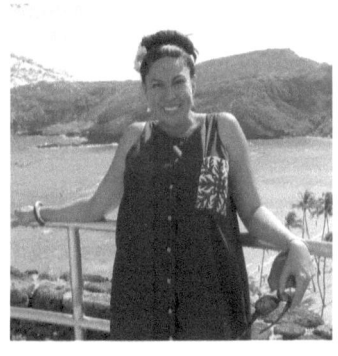

Leilani is the founder and director of 'Inana Healing, specializing in the design and implementation of progressive wellness environments. Leilani has studied Hawaiian Arts and Culture under Violet Ku'ulei Kahale Bourke for twenty-one years, honoring ancient traditions to create joy and vibrant health for a modern age.

'Inana Healing provides peak performance coaching, consulting, and delivery of direct services for international luxury spas and resorts, professional entertainment venues, and special populations. Leilani has recently launched Careshifters$_{tm}$ Healthy Aging Institute, serving the growing needs of the mature market.

You can reach Leilani on her website at www.inanahealing.com.

www.ingramcontent.com/pod-product-compliance
Lightning Source LLC
Chambersburg PA
CBHW020335290526
45785CB00005B/2031